Weight Loss

This Book Includes:

NLP for Fast Weight Loss

&

Weight Loss Motivation for Women

By James Adler & Elena Garcia

Copyright James Adler & Elena Garcia

Contents

Book 1
NLP for Fast Weight Loss
How to Lose Weight with Neuro-Linguistic Programming Techniques: Program Your Weight Loss Success NOW!

By James Adler

INTRODUCTION

It is my desire that this book will give you a general understanding of Neuro-Linguistic Programming and how you can use this method of study to lose weight and keep it off. Many people have little knowledge about this powerful discipline that allows you to change how you think. You will be empowered to achieve your weight loss goals.

This book introduces ideas and presents techniques exclusive to NLP. Neuro-linguistic Programming is sometimes referred to as "the study of success," and has assisted many people in reaching virtually any goal. It helped me to lose weight and keep it off. I know that it will assist you as well.

Most diet and exercise plans do not work because they do not utilize any techniques to change your mindset. The mind is where will power and motivation start. NLP techniques are centrally focused on the way that thought influences behavior. NLP makes it is possible to stay focused and motivated in order to achieve weight loss and, most importantly, to maintain it.

CHAPTER 1 PRACTICAL NLP FOR A BUSY PERSON IN THE 21ST CENTURY

Are you sick of the way that circumstances in your life have turned out, or even just the way that things are going? I have been there. I had goals, but would always fall short. A recurring question in the back of my mind was always, "There are others out there who are always winning; how can I win too?" I found out that the only thing I needed to do was change the way I looked at things, change the process that I used to deal with what happens. Success is not found in *what* happens to you, it is found in the way that you *handle* what happens. Find out how someone has achieved success and copy the techniques that they used to handle their circumstances. Neuro-linguistic Programming is just that simple.

Neuro-linguistic Programming has been proven to work for people who are looking to successfully solve a number of problems that they have encountered in life. Stress, anxiety, depression, phobias, addictions, relationship issues, difficulty with weight as experienced in eating disorders, and many other difficulties have been "cured" using Neuro-linguistic Programming strategies and techniques. The symptoms of these problems are not what need to be addressed. We need to determine how we ended up in these situations and change what steps we took to get there.

Neuro-linguistic Programming is not the study of *what* you think. It is the study of *how* you think. NLP looks into the process of thought and feeling. Practicing NLP techniques will change your behavior, which in turn, will change your outcome. It is easy to say, "Think positively," but without the tools to be able to do so, it is easier said than done. That is exactly what Neuro-linguistic Programming provided me with, the tools to think optimistically and confidently.

NLP looks at the connections linking how we think (neuro), communicate (linguistic) and the repetitions of our emotions and behaviors (programs). It is important to note the different parts of the terms in order to get the most out of the process.

The term "neuro" is referring to your neurological system. We come in contact with the world using the five senses. The information gathered through these senses is then communicated into conscious and unconscious thought. These thoughts trigger the neurological system which controls our bodily processes, behaviors, and sentiments.

"Linguistic" describes the way we employ language to understand the world around us, acquire and comprehend what happens to us in life, and the process in which we transfer that information to others.

The word "programming" is used to describe how we decipher, code, and store our experiences. Your personal programming consists of your internal processes and strategies (thinking patterns) that you use to make decisions, solve problems, learn, evaluate, and get results. NLP shows us how to recode our experiences and restructure our internal programming so that we can get the outcomes that we desire.

Modelling behavior is a key element of Neuro-linguistic Programming. The belief is that if one person can achieve success by following certain mental steps, then anyone can. Very simply, you ask someone who has attained success how they did it. You observe and listen to what they tell you. You use the answers as tools to apply to your own situation and follow the steps that they took. Questions like how they prepared for a certain situation or how they bounced back when having a set-back are examples that will help you in your circumstance.

Neuro-linguistic Programming is a toolkit full of useful techniques that you can use to study and attain success. There are hundreds of different techniques for different personalities and circumstances. They are all intended to help people succeed. It is usually recommended to learn about NLP through detailed books, from NLP practitioners and therapists, or take a seminar with a coach. The world of Neuro-linguistic Programming is vast. The more I studied, the more that there was to learn. The techniques can be used in any circumstance, for anyone. The possibilities of their results are endless.

Reaching and maintaining a healthy weight can be a difficult thing for some people to do. Failure leads to disappointment and shame. Sometimes these feelings lead to even more weight gain through over-eating or just lack of motivation to exercise. Eating disorders are another major hurdle to overcome in weight loss. You also need will power to exercise and resist the temptation to eat too much. I know I did. I successfully achieved a weight loss of thirty pounds and have continued to keep it off for the last five years, all by changing how I think. The understanding and use of Neuro-linguistic Programming strategies helped me and can help you as well.

Having a good comprehension of Neuro-linguistic Programming and its methods can lead success to every area of life. I will share with you how it helped me to achieve my goal of losing weight and maintaining that weight loss through a healthy diet and exercise.

CHAPTER 2: MIND OVER MATTER. GETTING STARTED ON NLP

Losing weight and keeping it off was always difficult for me. I knew *what* I needed to do. I just did not know *how* to mentally take steps to get there. A change of thinking and attitude toward myself, food, and exercise was required. I did not know how to make that adjustment. That is where Neuro-linguistic Programming came in. It gave me the tools that I needed in order to realize my goal by altering my thought processes and my feelings toward myself and food. I was able to lose weight and keep it off.

NLP is not a magic cure, but it will help you to reach your weight loss goals by changing the way that you think. In NLP we are given tools that enable us to be successful. Now, you are not going to lose weight with the power of your mind, but you will be able to change thoughts and behaviors that might hinder your weight loss. You will also develop attitudes and behaviors that will propel you in the right direction down the path to health! Our minds are very powerful and so is our imagination. Neuro-linguistic Programming helps us to use both to their full potential, assisting us in achieving and maintaining our goals.

With NLP, you can learn how to: make unhealthy habits undesirable and make heathy ones more desirable. You will be able to get rid of beliefs that may have kept you from your fitness goals and replace them with ones that will allow you to achieve healthy weight loss more easily.

Neuro-linguistic Programming tricks the mind into changing the way that it reacts to both unhealthy and healthy foods. You can instill new, positive behaviors while negating old, self-destructive behavior. Our minds can get rid of previously limiting beliefs and be programmed with new ones. How exciting!

How does this work? Well, NLP fools your mind into changing its response to certain stimuli. NLP also tricks the brain into believing things that we may not have thought to be true in the past. If you want a different mindset, NLP is your answer. Many people fail when it comes to losing weight and keeping it off. The most common reason for this is a negative or improper mind set. Here is some insight as to how our brains react to NLP methods when we first start to practice them. For example:

- The prefrontal cortex is the area of the brain that tells your body to pretend as if the healthy food you are consuming is delicious.

- Then the insula informs you that this is false. It brings up the same distasteful sensory information that you usually experience when eating health food.

- All of the sudden, your temporal and parietal lobes are acting strange. They are showing reflexive signs of pleasure!

- Now, the amygdala is sending out weak signals of pleasure to the other parts of the brain. These faint, pleasurable emotions signal the other areas to produce emotion. The better you fake it, the stronger you make it!

- Next, the hippocampus pairs up the feelings of pleasure with process of eating the healthy food. It tells the insula that you are in fact eating healthy food.

- This confirmation by the hippocampus changes the information in the insula. The insula now stores the new feelings connected to the healthy food and stores them away for future reference. You now have a new point of reference and new pathways in the brain!

The more we repeat these sorts of processes, the more feelings and ideas we can change. We can build many of new pathways in the brain. We can strengthen the effect of the NLP techniques by using them consistently. Soon enough, we will subconsciously have new ideas, emotions, and behaviors that will ensure our weight loss success.

Here are five tips that will help you to get the most out of NLP, enabling you to get the most out of your weight loss journey:

1. Model excellence. See what others who were/are successful in achieving weight loss have done or are doing. Choose a source that you trust; an example who's opinion that you respect. Do your research! In NLP we are taught that if another person can achieve a goal, we can too. Read and learn as much as possible about the person and technique that you are going to model. This will help you before you begin your program, and along the way!

2. Attitude is key! We need to take the time to prepare ourselves and set up a good foundation before starting out on our quest to achieve a goal. Before starting a new lifestyle we have to make sure that our outlook is positive, yet realistic. Realize that you will not know everything before you start. You will hit road blocks

along the way. You will have to move past obstacles. Just know above all else that you can do this! See yourself already fully engaged in your new lifestyle. Attitude is everything.

3. Be inquisitive and allow room for misunderstandings. You are not going to know everything ahead of time. Wondering about things (details or the big picture) will propel you to work harder to see how the process is going to play out. Curiosity will also push you to investigate and learn more about the NLP and how it benefits healthy eating and exercise. Misunderstandings will arise and at times you will get confused. This is ok, and can actually be quite beneficial. You will be pulled out of your comfort zone and forced into new ways of behaving and thinking.

4. Transformation is important. You will have to change. People want change in their lives but are unwilling to alter themselves and their behaviors. NLP techniques will help you to modify your thought processes and get rid of past behavior that may have been leading you down a path that you did not want to be on. By utilizing NLP techniques, you can put the past behind you, including mistakes and negative thought processes. You can start to anticipate positive outcomes. Embrace the transformations and modifications with open arms.

5. Make the most of the journey by having a blast! Your road to weight loss does not just end in one concrete location. There are many twists and turns on the path. With so many outcomes and so many different avenues that will help you achieve weight loss, you might as well choose the fun road, instead of the high road. It has been proven that people stick with programs that are enjoyable, and what is more enjoyable than FUN? Be serious about losing weight, but learn to laugh at yourself. Take the journey seriously, but taking yourself too seriously may sabotage your program! Enjoy the process!

The first thing I did when I began down the road to successful weight loss was to make sure that I had plenty of motivation. Motivation is a driving force in achieving any goal. We all know it definitely takes motivation to get to the gym and work out. Exercise is a large part of the solution to staying healthy and losing weight. I took certain steps using a visualization technique that helped to encourage my desire to work out and reach my goal. I had to be enthusiastic about starting my journey and this technique helped me to do so. It can help you as well!

VISUALIZATION TECHNIQUE

Step 1- Take the time to relax. Breathe deeply and unwind without distraction. Close your eyes and stand up.

Step 2- Allow yourself to think about a time in the imminent future when you will be delighted with yourself because you have been going to the gym and exercising on a regular basis.

Step 3- Visualize as an outsider how you will look when you have been working out consistently. How do you appear physically? Are you the size you want to be? You are toned and looking confident and happy. In your mind envision every detail of your new appearance.

Step 4- Take an actual step forward and picture yourself stepping into your new self. You will now be visualizing everything through your own eyes, this "new you." You are physically fit and feeling amazing.

Step 5- Be conscious of how spectacular it feels to be in shape. Realize how much energy and motivation you have now that you have achieved success. What does it feel like to be in your healthy, fit body?

Step 6- What are you noticing with your five senses? What emotional feelings are you experiencing? Turn these feelings up, like an emotional volume control. Feel them to the extreme. Allow yourself to feel incredible in the most intense way while you visualize yourself going to the gym or getting ready to work out. Revel in this moment for as long as possible.

Step 7- Hold on to those emotions as you come back to your current self and open your eyes.

When I directed my thoughts in a certain way I was able to motivate myself to exercise. This is because the central nervous system does not recognize a real event or an imagined event as dissimilar. What you visualize in your mind can be more powerful than what you tell yourself. The imagination is more influential than the conscious psyche.

BELIEF CREATION

Do you feel like you are stuck in your old belief system regarding your fitness or weight loss goals? Well, you can change that despite what you may think. It is easy to do. We are not stuck in our thinking. We need to make new beliefs and give ourselves more options and flexibility. Otherwise, our outcome will never change. You can never get something that you have never had by doing the same things you have always done.

An example of my own use of Belief Creation had to do with my own physical fitness, or should I say lack thereof. I created the belief that I could get through a rigorous workout without too much effort... and without dying of course. When I began to honestly believe it, guess what? I WAS ABLE TO DO IT! Just believing that I could get through a super intense workout made it easy for me to make progress and accomplish something I had never done before. My negative, self-sabotaging beliefs had been holding me back!

Practice creating small beliefs first. This will enable you to erase doubt about the fact that this kind of technique will work at all. Beliefs cannot be created when there is uncertainty involved. The more that you see this method work, the greater the impact your newly created beliefs.

Here is an easy way to integrate Belief Creation, step by step, into your weight loss program:

1. Focus on something that you truly believe. Make sure that it is something you sincerely know to be factual. It could be as simple as, "The world is round." Whatever belief you choose, visualize it. What image do you see? Where is the location of the image? Centered? Left? Right? Is it near or far in your mind's eye? Is there any self-talk associated with this image, any sounds? After analyzing and noting these things, focus your thoughts on something else. It could be anything: laundry, the rain, your recently stubbed toe, etc. You can also let your brain relax and think about nothing.

2. Ok, now it is time to choose a belief that you do not truly believe in. Choosing a belief that you do not really care if it is true or false may be most helpful. Follow the questioning process as in step one, while visualizing this belief.

3. Now that you have figured out where the two visualizations of these ideas/beliefs are, pick a belief that you would like to realize as truth. For example,

"Healthy, alkaline foods are delicious." Bring up this belief in your mind's eye. Take note of where the location is of this image. First, shift this newfound belief into the same spot where you had the belief that you do not really care about. Next, move the new belief to the same spot that you placed your validated belief. If you have any words (self-talk) or sounds associated with the new belief, say them over and over to yourself as you park the picture into the validated idea position.

Some issues that you may encounter:

- The new picture/image will not shift into a new position. All that you must do to fix this problem is to put the picture far into the distance, away from you, until it is almost out of sight. When it is almost too small to see, bring it back close to you. Place it where it should be, in the same spot that you hold the belief that you see as fact.

If the picture you hold in regard to your freshly created belief keeps moving back to where it was when you originally came up with it, you can:

- Make a sound in your head to signal the movement of the image to its new "believed" spot.

- Picture yourself putting glue on the back of the picture and stick it into its new position.

- Imagine yourself staple-gunning or nailing the image where you want it to stay.

- Envision any way that you would keep something in a relocated spot in real life, and fix your image using that method.

- Note: make sure that all images are equal size, especially the believed image and the newly created belief image.

Make sure that your new belief will work. You can do this by letting your mind attach to a different thought, or just let it relax and go blank for a bit. Now, think about the belief that you created. What position did it automatically move to? Is it the same size as the others? Does your self-talk believe it to be true?

If it is still not working, keep doing the exercise over and over, from start to finish, until it works. This method is a simple and effective way to create a new belief that will get your weight loss program off to a great start.

MAPPING ACROSS

When we begin any sort of a new program in our lives, it is sometimes important for us to change our view of certain things. If we decide that something makes us happy, or that certain foods are delicious, it makes our new lifestyle much easier to adopt and adapt to. In my life, I needed to change the way that I felt about raw, green vegetables or I was not going to get far in my healthy weight loss venture. I needed to feel the same way for vegetables that I did for French fries and tortilla chips! Sound impossible? It is not. This method can also work for addictions or compulsions, such as a sugar addiction. Here is how you can see things differently and experience a fondness for things that you may have never thought to be possible:

1. Figure out exactly what idea you would like to alter. You will need to mentally put yourself directly into this situation. Let us go back to my example. In my mind I was seated in front of a huge table full of dark, green, raw vegetables. I could see them, smell them, and hear the awful crunching noise that they made in my mouth. YUCK! I took detailed notes of the sights, sounds, and smells associated with the situation. When you write down what you notice in your situation, do not be afraid to have too many details. Also, take note of where the

mental image is playing out in your mind. Where is it, how bright is it, and how large is it?

2. Next, picture yourself in a situation that brings a large amount of pleasure or joy. It could also be a situation that you disgusts you. If you are addicted to ice cream and want to be rid of that feeling, visualize a sewer or something revolting. To make it easy for myself, I envisioned sitting in front of a large dessert tray, filled with every sweet, delicious cake, cookie, and pastry I could imagine. I noted every detail, as in the first step, and relished in the moment!

3. You want to note the differences in the situations. What answers to the questions that you asked yourself are almost opposite? You may only find a couple, but these are very important. It could be as simple as one scenario playing out in color and the other in black and white.

4. Now, you want to use at least one of the differences and apply it to the first situation (the feeling that you want to change or get rid of). For instance, in my first visualization the size was rather small, and the room was cold and dank. The colors were pretty dull. In the second, it was a large scene in a warm room full of color and lovely smells. All I had to do was visualize myself sitting in front of the vegetables and switch up certain

aspects of the scene. I made the visualization huge, imagined the room warm and colorful, and full of delicious smells. I would repeat this over and over, taking breaks after each switch. Eventually, I did not have to consciously make the switch at all!

It really is that simple. Mapping Across works. I hope that you will see the importance in this technique and apply it to your own weight loss program. It has a wide variety of uses and will have a huge impact on your state of mind!

BEHAVIOR CREATOR

"When you fail to prepare, prepare to fail." Taking the time to set things up for yourself before you jump into a new, healthy, fit lifestyle is of the utmost importance. Mental imagery techniques allow us to lay the ground work that will help us to successfully achieve our weight loss goals and live a healthy lifestyle.

I found mental imagery helpful in making sure that I did not skip meals. I had heard that it was very important to eat 5 or 6 mini-meals throughout the day, and I had issues even sticking to 3. Others have used mental imagery to motivate themselves to work out harder and more often. I encourage you to use mental imagery to change whatever behavior it is that you believe will make a large impact on your weight loss program. Keep in mind though that more often than not little changes can have a powerful effect.

There are many types of mental imagery techniques, but the Behavior Creator will help with many issues that you have, or events that you might like to prevent, while getting started on your weight loss venture. It will help you to enact a new behavior subconsciously so that you do not have to expend energy *consciously* making a continual effort. You be able to operate more efficiently this way.

If we want new behaviors to stick around, we must connect the behavior to the outcome that we desire; which in this case is weight loss. If we can connect the end result with a new behavior, it is easier to keep it going. Here is how you can create a new behavior that will ensure your success in your weight loss program.

1. Choose a type of behavior that you want to develop. Pick one that is going to help you achieve your fitness

goals. For me, it was to make sure that I ate many meals throughout the day. Others have decided to make exercise their focus. Do what works best for you.

2. Create a visualization of the behavior and how a situation might play out while you are engaged in it. See yourself fully engaged in the newly created behavior. Watch the visualization as if you were watching a movie. You can be the star, or watch someone else performing the said action that you have created. Use your imagination and make the scene your own. Observe every detail.

3. If you are visualizing someone else engaging in this behavior, put yourself into their role. After watching them play the part, take over and observe yourself participating from an outside perspective.

4. Now, feel yourself behaving in such a manner. How is your body moving? What muscles are you using? Are you tense or relaxed? What is your posture like?

We must test this behavior to make sure it works and is really instilled into our subconscious.

1. Create 4 scenarios in your mind where this behavior will be of use. These situations should be ones that would have normally prompted your old behavior.

2. Place yourself in the scene. Sense everything that is going on around you. You are there in the moment. Take note of everything that is being picked up by your 5 senses.

3. Did your behavior change this time? Did you engage in your new behavior as opposed to your old, unwanted behavior? If you are still stuck in your old behavior, repeat the steps above to solidify the new behavior. Keep testing until you automatically use your newly created behavior.

CHAPTER 3 NLP During Your Weight Loss Program

Thanks to a boosted motivation level, I was on my way to the "new me." At the beginning of the process I realized that every day I felt as if I was battling my old eating habits. I would over eat. Consuming more calories than I was burning was stifling my goal. Eating the wrong foods was also keeping me from achieving physical wellbeing. I used a specific technique to change my bad eating habits. It is referred to as the Swish Pattern.

The Swish Pattern is a useful tool in changing old bad habits easily. It is a technique where you replace an undesirable habit for one you would prefer to have. I wanted to replace my unhealthy eating habits (junk food and over-eating) with healthy eating habits (energy foods and eating healthy portions). This tool helped me to change my thoughts and thought process regarding these habits, which in turn changed the bad behavior.

SWISH PATTERN

First, choose the habit/behavior that you desire to replace. Visualize it in your mind. Be in the moment of acting out this behavior. Use your five senses to recognize exactly what it feels like. What emotions do you have? Isolate a certain, vividly detailed image of yourself in the midst of engaging in this habit. For me, it was imagining myself shoving pizza into my mouth. Make sure you recognize that /this is something you have done in the past and that you want to keep it there. Take a mental picture.

Next, using all of your senses again, create another image of yourself being successful by replacing that bad eating habit with a healthy one. This will be your replacement snap shot. It is vivid, intense, and vibrant. In mine, I had eaten well and used proper portions. I was healthy and energized thanks to making good choices in regard to food. I stepped outside of this picture to see myself in it. At the bottom corner of the new image, you will place a tiny version of yourself in the midst of your bad habit. This tiny picture is dark and colorless.

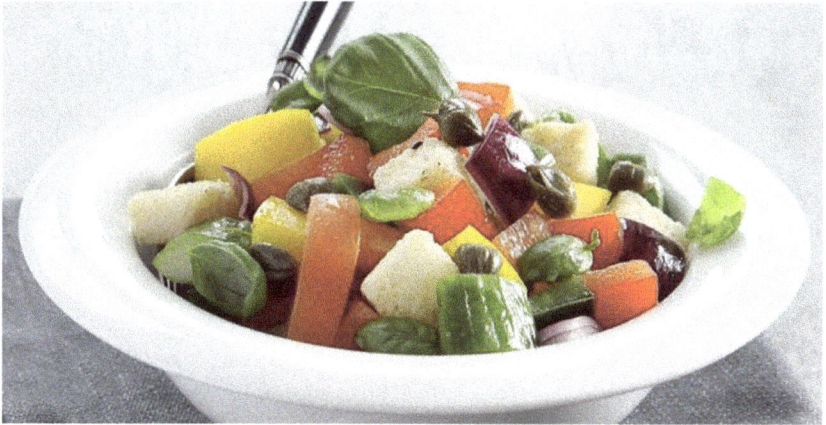

A Healthy and Balanced Meal or...

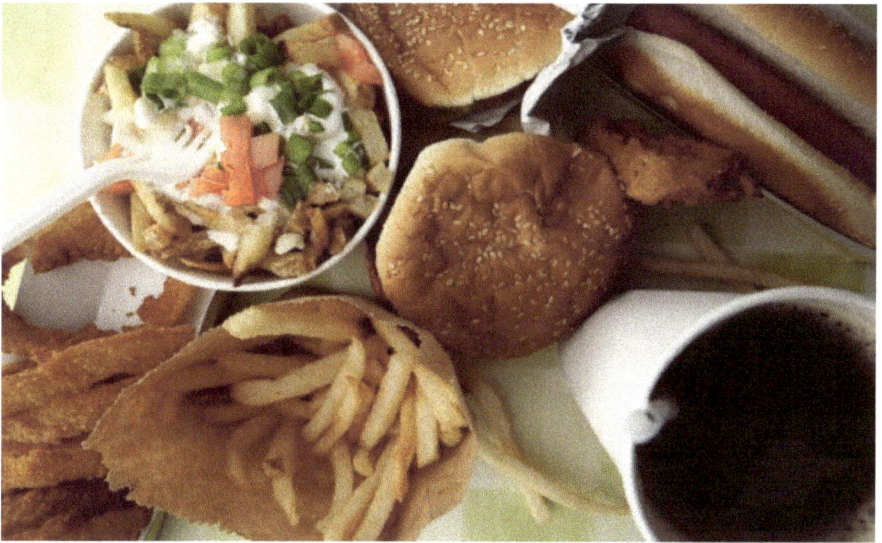

Indulging in Unhealthy Habits...?

Now, re-visualize the first picture, the old you. At the bottom corner, darken the future picture (of you and your replacement behavior) and make it small. You can still see it but it is darker. Put yourself back into the poor emotional state that you are currently in. This is currently the big image. You should be feeling all of the self-defeating emotions associated with your bad habit like disappointment and self-loathing. Fully connect yourself with that moment.

Next, instantaneously switch the two images. Bring back the "new you," with your replacement behavior. Make it huge and colorful, full of everything to stimulate your senses. Shrink the picture of your unwanted behavior at the same time, moving it back into the corner and darken it. When you do this, make a "swwwwwisssssssshhhhhhhhh" sound. As I did this I would mentally jump into the replacement behavior image. The picture of you in the future is now the present. The old behavior is in the past, exactly where you want it to be.

I repeated this several times. Switching the pictures and jumping into my new behavioral image while "swooshing." Gradually increase the speed of the switch. Each time I was doing it faster and faster. Eventually it will become instantaneous. Replacing your bad eating habit will be as simple as that.

SETTING AN ANCHOR

Another Neuro-linguistic Programming technique I used on a consistent basis during my weight loss journey was Anchoring. Setting an anchor was immensely beneficial to me and I hope that it is for you as well. It helped me to get back the feeling of being motivated, healthy and happy like I used to be when I was in shape and healthy years ago. This technique helped to keep me driven during my weight loss program. The beauty of this process is that if one anchor does not produce the results you are looking for, it can always be replaced.

Anchoring Facts:

- They can be produced artificially or naturally (due to events).

- They can occur because of a single emotionally charged event or subconsciously through repetition, for example: advertising.

- Needs to be repeated; it can fade with time.

- Make sure you set the anchor when the feeling you want to reinforce is at its peak.

- Choose a very intense memory.

- Make sure that the stimulus you are using is as exclusive as possible. Don't use something you do all of the time.

- I stacked (set) my anchors for approximately 30 minutes; the longer the duration of repetition the better.

1. Choosing a memory- I remembered a time I was at the gym and was asked to be a trainer because I was at my physical best. You choose your own. Make sure it was emotionally intense.

2. Reliving the memory- Associate yourself with the memory. Be in that moment and see it through your own eyes. This made my feelings more intense. I made the picture of the event extremely colorful, large and bright. I intensified my feelings to the maximum.

3. Anchoring the memory- When I felt my emotions at their peak, I pinched the back of my hand. That was my trigger. You can do whatever works best for you: rub your earlobe, grab your knee, etc.

4. Stop at your peak- Release your trigger when your emotion peaks. I had to practice this step a few times before I had it down.

5. Testing the trigger/anchor- I stopped for a while and thought about something else, then used my trigger. If anchoring was successful, it will bring you directly back to that lovely emotional state immediately.

6. Repeat. - Repeat this several times. To make my anchor stronger and more powerful, I set 3-4 memories of times when I felt the same way to that identical trigger.

Anchoring was the most effective way to put myself in a motivated, positive mind set during my weight loss program. I used it almost every day, throughout the day. My trigger helped me be able to feel awesome and driven on demand. What better way to make it through a weight loss program?

SELF-CHECK

An additional way I used NLP ideas in my weight loss program was to check in with myself every day. I needed to make sure that I was staying on track. I would think about and ask myself these key questions:

1. What do I desire?
2. How will getting that help me?

3. What obstacles are keeping me from getting it?
4. What is essential to me?
5. What is working best in this situation?
6. What could be enhanced?
7. What resources am I going to utilize?

Self-evaluation is necessary to achieve any goal. Success in the short or long term requires that questions be asked and answers be evaluated. Then, if necessary, redirection must occur.

DISENGAGING A COMPULSION

I, as many people do, suffered from an eating disorder that some people do not recognize as one. Binge eating was a serious issue for me. I would engorge myself and end up feeling sick, physically and emotionally. I would feel great while I was committing the crime, but the aftermath left me feeling disgusting. I always hated myself afterward.

I used the following steps to break myself of this horrible compulsion. It worked very well for me. I have not fallen into doing it again thanks to this very beneficial process.

- First, I figured out what type of food I liked to binge on. For me, it was fast food; any type of fast food. For some it may be candy, carbs, etc.

- Next, I focused on the situation in which I would normally use this behavior. For me it was at the end of the month after working long hours. I would use it to reward myself, but it was really a punishment of sorts. Actually, it got so bad that I would automatically do it without even thinking about it. You must figure out in what situations you tend to binge.

- Picture the circumstances in your mind. Use your five senses to notice what is going on around you. I paid special attention to the actual food I was eating. Details are key.

- Clear your mind of the entire scene for a few moments. I would imagine a blank blue screen.

- Imagine next something that repulses you. For me, it was a decaying dead animal with maggots all over it. It can be garbage, vomit, or feces; anything that makes you sick. Imagine the taste and smell of it in your mouth. I would feel as though I was going to vomit. I used all of my senses again in this exercise. See it, smell it, hear it, taste it, and feel it.

- Remove the image from your mind once again and go back to imagining your binging situation. During your session this time, notice how pleasurable it is. When you take a bite this time around, you should notice that the sense of tasting something horrible has overwhelmed you. Exactly like when you were experiencing whatever it is that disgusts you.

- Do this five to ten times.

- Clear your mind once again for a few moments.

- Finally, imagine binging on your favorite food. This round should not bring about the same pleasure and desire. Personally, I just felt sick. I was experiencing the negative emotions I had in regard to the dead animal while picturing myself eating pizza; that which used to bring me pleasure.

I was able to be successful in disengaging my compulsive, automatic binge eating by using this method. It was a relief to never have to feel out of control again. I was cured and felt empowered once more.

COGNITIVE REFRAMING

Sometimes we make things more difficult for ourselves than they need to be. If we just take a little time and change our words for certain things, sometimes we can change our entire thought process. When we use Cognitive Reframing, we are choosing to cut off a negative way of thinking and talking; replacing these thoughts, phrases, and words with more positive ones. This not only works for weight loss and exercise regimes, but has been proven effective in many other areas. Even major corporations have used this method in dealing with customers and employees.

When used to your advantage, Cognitive Reframing can help you to turn a situation where you do not feel empowered into a moment of empowerment. This is a perfect way to change the way you think about weight loss and food, while in the midst of your program. Come up with your own language for your weight loss *journey*... see what I did there. It is that easy!

When you have a weight loss program that you are implementing, it is easy to get stressed out. Any major change in life can bring stress, but a new weight loss routine can be very intense because we are changing our entire lifestyle. We are causing stress to our mind and our bodies. We are basically shocking our entire system and it is very taxing. It is this stress that we put on ourselves that will usually thwart our weight loss efforts, not laziness or hunger. Cutting carbs, calories, and exerting extra physical energy by working out is physically and mentally demanding for anyone; from the beginner to the experienced.

Here are some more idea to get you started:
- "Calorie counting" BECOMES "Meal design"
- "Cheat day/cheat meal" BECOMES "Flexible eating plan/plateau breaker"
- "Diet" BECOMES "Modified eating regimen"
- "Difficult workout" BECOMES "High intensity"
- "Weight lifting" BECOMES "Strength training"
- "Will-power" BECOMES "Skill-power"
- "Lose weight" BECOMES "Burn fat"

As you can see, it really is that easy! Here are some steps you can take to come up with your own positive language and reframe your own thinking:

1. **Do a little research.** Figure out what negative thought processes you have in regard to your weight loss. Learn how pessimists see things. Read up on negative and positive explanatory thinking. It will help you to figure out what to change in order to have a more positive outlook so that you can keep stress to a minimum.

2. **Pay attention to what and how you are thinking.** Observe when you become stressed and what negative thoughts you might be experiencing at the time. Being mindful about what you are thinking can help. See your thoughts and thought processes from the outside; observe your own thinking. You will get better and better at sensing these thoughts when they first come to mind. Then, you can start to turn them around when they come about. You will go from negative to positive thinking easily with just a little bit of practice. Soon it will be effort less, and you will find losing weight to be much less stressful!

3. **Now that you are aware of your negative thought processes in regard to weight loss, test them.** A major component of reframing requires us to check for the validity of our thoughts. Are they real? Are they true? If they are, figure out a more positive way to

look at what is happening. No, you are not lying to yourself. You will simply be seeing things more positively, allowing you to have a less stressful experience in general. Constantly try to see things differently, in a more positive light.

4. **Now it is time to consciously switch your thoughts.** Now that you: know the effects of negative and how they affect your stress levels, are able to label negative thoughts as they arise, have checked to make sure they are valid, and have looked at weight loss in a more positive way, it is time to switch your thoughts. Any negative thoughts that you have in regard to your weight loss program can bring about negative emotions and stress. Simply come up with new key phrases that are positive to replace the old, negative ones. The more you use this new motivating, uplifting language, the less stressful and more positive your weight loss journey will be! It really is all in your head!

LAST STRAW METHOD

In order to pursue a goal, especially an all-encompassing or difficult one, we need motivation. Motivation not only gives us a jump start that we need to begin achieving our goals, it also is the main thing that keeps us going in the right direction during the process. This technique helps us to take an unpleasant emotion or habit and blow it up until we cannot tolerate it any longer. It makes you feel like, "ENOUGH IS ENOUGH!!" This method really helped me to put my foot down... with myself.

This method helps us to take something that is not healthy or positive, and say, "I have had enough!" Get rid of things that are not in your best interest with this technique. Most of us are guilty of tolerating things that we should not just because they may not be detrimental to our existence. In regard to weight loss, this could be midnight binging on cookies. It could be the soda on our break at work, or the occasional de-stressing cigarette. Yet, even though these things are not good for us, they are not unendurable. A lot of the time we need an insufferable circumstance in order to put an end to it.

This is where the Last Straw Method is useful. It allows us to alter our thinking and make our mind believe that the situation or habit has become unbearable. This is known as a threshold pattern. We must not only get to the threshold, we must go over it.

Here is an example of reaching your threshold: After binging on pizza all night, the night before, you woke up disappointed in yourself and appalled by your own behavior. Yet, you did not stop the binging. Two days later you polished off a gallon of ice cream and a 2 lb bag of fries.

Here is an example of going over your threshold: Your boyfriend calls you fat and "moos" every time you eat. You are distraught and dump him.

Here is put the Last Straw Method into practice:

Visualize a situation when you were *at* your threshold, but did not go over it.

As the intensity of the situation builds, take note of all the details that you can. Are noises becoming slowly louder or quieter? Is the picture of the situation getting larger, smaller, dimmer, or brighter? How is the vision changing as the tension is building?

Now, visualize a situation where you went *over* the threshold. Usually the visualization will undergo a massive change when you cross the threshold. Did you see another picture that was very different from the one you saw before crossing the threshold? Did you hear self-talk saying "I'm done" or "no more?" How did you look? Did you appear happier or more self-assured?

The last thing that you need to do is apply the feelings and sensory information that you picked up on in your "crossing the threshold" scenario, and apply them to your "reaching the threshold" scenario. Visualize the whole scene differently, with more confidence.

Push yourself over the edge and never deal with the same issue again! Repeat as many times as you need to in order to feel that, "ENOUGH IS ENOUGH!"

FUTURE PACING

One of the best ways that I have found to curb my appetite using NLP, is through Future Pacing. In this technique, we use mental pictures and visualizations (I think of them as movies in my head) to make changes in ourselves that we will need to access in the future. We can use anchors to bring about the new feeling when needed.

We can test this technique by triggering the anchor and seeing if the newly programmed thought or idea kicks in. It should arise automatically. Here is a practical, easy way to use this technique:

Visualize yourself in a situation where you want to engage in a certain behavior or would like to end up with a certain outcome. For me I chose being at a party with a lot of high calorie snacks, high fat deserts and h'ordeuvres, and drinks. I do not eat any of them. Not only because I have self-control, but because I was just not hungry!! Pretend like you are watching a movie. What are you wearing, doing, and saying? What smells do you smell? How do you sound? As I stayed away from the no-no foods, I was confident. I could see it in my posture and the way I walked. I was not shaken by the food.

Now, jump into the picture and experience the situation first hand. What can you hear, see, and feel? Note everything about the experience you are having while utilizing your new trait.

When you feel the new behavior peak, or become the strongest, use a physical trigger and anchor the feeling to it. I usually tap my palm, but do whatever works best for you.

Practice and relate your new characteristic to all of the sensory information that you picked up while visualizing the scenario playing out in your head. All of the things that you saw, smelled, felt, heard, etc., should now bring about the new behavior or emotion that you wanted to enact within yourself. Do not forget to use your trigger. After rehearsing many times, anchoring the feeling, and observing everything around you with all of your senses, you experience this new conduct in real life situations, exactly how you experienced it in your visualization.

COMPULSION BLOWOUT TECHNIQUE

Do you have a compulsion that you feel might be out of your control? Is this behavior inhibiting your weight loss in any way? If so, the Compulsion Blowout Technique may be the perfect option to help you get rid of unnecessary, compulsive behavior.

This technique worked perfectly for me. I used it to rid myself of my chocolate "addiction." Anytime I thought of chocolate, smelled chocolate, or saw chocolate, I ate it. Even my co-workers' candy dishes and my son's Halloween stash were not safe from my compulsive chocolate eating. Today, I am in control. Not that I *never* eat chocolate, but I dictate when and where I consume it. Here is how you can join me in beating compulsive behavior:

Picture the one thing you have a huge weakness for: smoking, fatty foods, carbs, candy, etc. Pay attention to where this mental picture is in your mind. Is it directly in the middle of your mind? Is it near, far, to the left, or to the right? How large is it?

Now picture one thing that relates to a behavior that is non-compulsive for you. For example, taking vitamins, or brushing your hair. Where is the image? What size is it? Ask yourself the same questions as in number one and note your answers.

If it is helpful for you, list all of the answers on a piece of paper. One set for the thing that represents your compulsion and the other for the non-compulsive image. List the differences in what you see and hear. Note the dissimilarities.

Now, start playing around with the image in your mind related to your compulsive behavior. You want to increase the size, location, or sounds related to that image. For instance, if the size of the image is a lot larger than the other, keep blowing it up in your mind until it is so undeniably huge that it is no longer a compulsion for you. You want the image to morph into one that is absolutely ridiculous. If there is a sound involved, turn up the volume in your mind until it seems to blow out your eardrums. This will disallow the compulsive behavior from having any control over you anymore. Say you see a chocolate bar, blow it up until it is so large that you get a stomach ache just visualizing it.

Do this quite a few times, in the same exact manner. Take breaks, but go back to the same process. Visualize it, and then quickly exaggerate!

Test your method and see if the change sticks. With a little work it will. Soon enough, your mind will switch up the image automatically and you will not fall victim to your compulsion anymore!

CHAPTER 4 NLP to Maintain Weight Loss Success

Once I achieved victory in losing weight through diet and exercise, I realized that I still had one more part to my goal. I wanted to be successful in maintaining the "new me." In evaluating this secondary goal, I realized that it was actually just as challenging, if not more difficult than successfully losing the weight in the first place.

Maintaining a healthier, thinner self is a long, slow process. Self-control is used on a regular basis and motivation must always be there to exercise. I was happy with myself, and that helped to encourage me. The amount of time that I had spent implementing and developing new habits was also advantageous in retaining my weight loss. Yet, because I had lost weight years before and gained it back, I knew the possibility of it happening again would always be there.

This time around, I took an extra step to ensure my long-term weight loss success. Neuro-linguistic Programming helped me to make certain that I would not gain weight again. It was extremely beneficial to continue utilizing the same tools I used during my program of weight loss to maintain my newfound health and figure. The same tools that helped me to drop the pounds assisted me in keeping them off. I added one more technique to my arsenal to make sure that I would be able to maintain my lighter, healthier self: a Well Formed Outcome.

A Well Formed Outcome helped me to keep the weight off by reminding me of and helping me to focus on my goal. My goal was to be lean and healthy, not just to lose weight and end up gaining it again. Sure, I had been triumphant in dropping the pounds. However, by having a Well Formed Outcome, I was able to ensure that I would stay motivated for the long-term in order to stay leaner and healthy.

Well Formed Outcomes are usually developed when you begin pursuing a goal. Yet, it is also what will keep you going until the end. It will aid you and be a driving force in staying successful when used as a long-term motivation tool.

Here are some tips that I used to create my Well Formed Outcome:

1) Understand *what* you want, not what you *do not* want.

Goals must have a positive focus. Instead of wanting to lose weight or not be fat; a better goal would be, "I would like to be healthy and trim." Focus on something you want to have instead of what you would like to stay away from.

2) Have a decent time frame.

Give yourself enough time to get the job done. Do not be too vague. Saying that I would like to lose 30 pounds as soon as possible might have been too overwhelming for me. Deciding to be healthy and trim is great, but without a time frame at all, it would have been harder to track and monitor my progress. "I would like to become healthy and trim in a year and stay that way for the rest of my life." This goal is both positive and gives a decent amount of time to accomplish that it.

3) Make sure to take full responsibility.

I was solely responsible for my outcome. No one else can be used as an excuse for why goals cannot be reached. This is not to say that you may not need help along the way, but no one else can be blamed for failure.

4) Focus and be specific with your outcome.

Utilizing all of my senses, I sat down and focused. I wrote out in detail how I would feel once I achieved my goal. The more specific that the details are, the more powerful the aspiration to succeed will be.

5) What resources are necessary to be successful and reach the objective?

What information will I need? What gear must I buy? What other resources can help me to reach my goal? These are all important questions to note and answer. Knowing where I wanted to go and how I was going to get there helped to motivate me.

6) Go over your goals on a regular basis.

Goals must be imbedded into the subconscious. Remember, the subconscious cannot tell when something is an actual event or when it is imaginary. Everyday feel your future success as if you are already there experiencing it for yourself.

Adapting the techniques that I used during my weight loss program to my maintenance program helped me to hold on to my thinner self. Additionally, creating my future success and reliving it in my mind everyday was a powerful tool in maintaining my weight loss. I was able to concentrate on being fit and healthy, instead of falling back into negative behaviors. I am still incredibly motivated five years later, all thanks to Neuro-linguistic Programming methods.

CONCLUSION

Thank you again for purchasing this book!

I hope this book was able to help you see that Neuro-linguistic Programming is an immensely useful field of study that will enable you to reach your weight loss goals. Disappointment and shame will be a thing of the past. Achievement is in your future, do not delay. The "new you" is waiting!

Staying healthy is the most important thing that you can do for yourself. It takes motivation, will power and hard work but is a most rewarding venture to undertake. Most people do not realize that it is the power of the mind that controls the body. Harness and redirect the power of yours. Literally, it is all in your head.

Imagine never "yo-yo" dieting again. Picture yourself desiring to go to the gym and enjoying working out. Your imagination will be a driving force in helping you reach these goals. I know my mother would always tell me to use my imagination as a child, but I never thought it could be such a mighty tool.

NLP has helped many people to be successful, and it helped me to reach my goals as well. NLP is a vital tool for anyone who is trying to lose weight. How can you go wrong using techniques derived from "the study of success?" Failure will no longer be an option.

I wish you well on your quest to lose weight. You can do it! I did.

Finally, I would like to ask you to do me a little favor and comment on my book on Amazon.
Thank you and good luck with your NLP journey!

James

www.YourWellnessBooks.com

ALKALINE-PALEO SUPERFOODS FOR OPTIMAL NUTRITION

Tips & Recipes to Help You Thrive!

- NATURAL WEIGHT LOSS
- MORE ENERGY FOR LIFE

ELENA GARCIA & JAMES ADLER

Free Complimentary eBook to Help You on Your Journey:

Sign up for free at: www.YourWellnessBooks.com/newsletter

Book 2

Weight Loss Motivation
for Women
Change Your Mindset, Stop Torturing Yourself with Perfectionism, and Create Super Healthy Habits You Enjoy

by Elena Garcia

Disclaimer

A physician has not written the information in this book. It is advisable that you visit a qualified dietician so that you can obtain a highly personalized treatment for your case, especially if you want to lose weight effectively. This book is for informational and educational purposes only and is not intended for medical purposes. Please consult your physician before making any drastic changes to your diet.

Chapter 1 Life is a Balancing Act

Who wants to feel better and look better? What woman doesn't, right? I hear women **EVERYDAY** and **EVERYWHERE** saying, "as soon as I have more time", "as soon as the new year starts", "as soon as I have more money", "as soon as the kids are back in school", "as soon as I feel better... Then, I'm going to start dieting and exercising and taking better care of myself!"

Well, guess what? Those days we pretend are lingering out there in the future are not coming. Those are excuses we make all the time that keep us from being the healthiest, strongest women we can be. Because women's lives are so busy and we spend so much of our time nurturing others, we have a full arsenal of excuses to combat our own efforts at maintaining our own wellbeing. There is no better day than today to start making simple changes that will make you feel and look so much better. You've taken a first step by opening this book and admitting that your lifestyle could use some healthy changes!

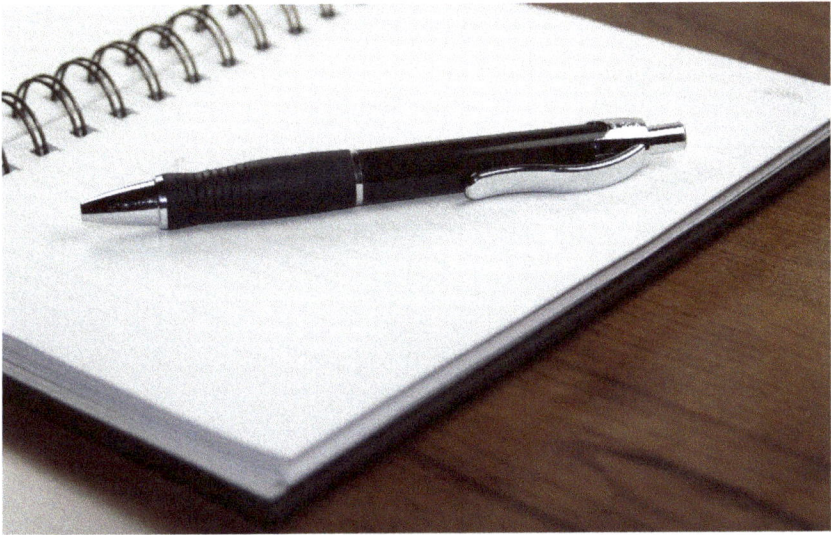

Take one more important first step with me and reflect on where you are right now:

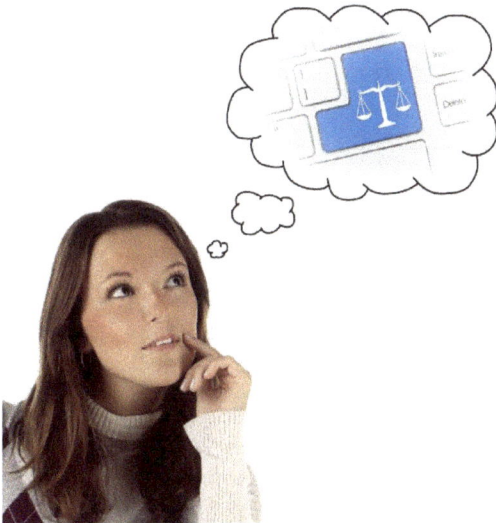

-Are you overweight?

-Do you need to lose just a few pounds, or do you need to shed 20 or more pounds in order to be healthy?

-Do you want to have more energy and feel better in general?

-Do you have a healthy diet but need more physical activity to become stronger?

-Are you in good shape but know you have some unhealthy habits that are holding you back?

-Do you need to find more quiet moments in your day for reflection and planning?

If you answered yes to any of these questions, keep reading! Just a few small changes in your day will reap huge dividends in the effort to become the best and healthiest version of yourself. The most important thing is- be honest with yourself. In order to get where you want, you need to know where you are, right? You can be honest, realistic and positive. This is what this book is all about...

Women in general are perfectionist. We compare ourselves to what we believe to be the ideal woman, and when we fall short of that ideal, we beat ourselves up and we give up. There is no perfect woman. She is a myth. I call it: deceptive marketing. They sell us this image to make us buy more and more products, ranging from beauty & fashion to weight loss pills, unrealistic cleanses, change your life in 7 days programs or be perfect in 3 easy steps. This is what clever marketers do. They create images of perfection that stay in our subconscious mind. Let's be real- there is no such thing as perfection. Of course, I am not saying we should not strive for progress, we should. But first of all we need to overcome guilt-trips and chasing something that is not real.

Still want to believe there are perfect women? Point out those women you think are perfect, the ones you believe have it all, and I promise it doesn't take long to identify the flaws and burdens that they carry. Stop comparing yourself to other women – the only woman you have to be better than is the one you were yesterday! Focus on where you are today and what your goals are for a more healthful lifestyle, a lifestyle that you deserve. Reject everything that doesn't support you in your goals, including unrealistic expectations or deceptive marketing. You can be the best you can, just by switching off all those images of perfection and focusing on yourself; your self-love and intuition.

PERFECTION-NO

FOCUS ON PROGRESS

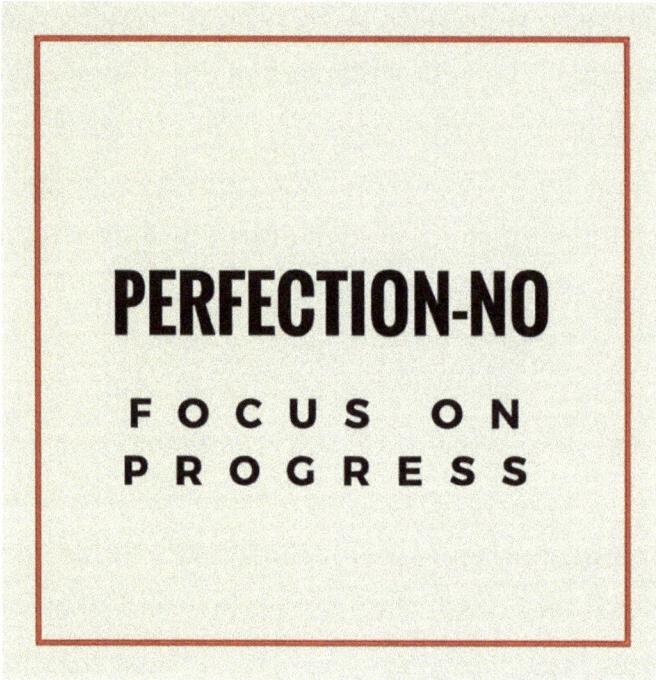

Another misconception we train ourselves with that stems from our perfectionism is believing we don't deserve the time it would take to become healthy. Women are guilt mongers. We feel guilt over everything. How many times have you told yourself, "I'm not a good enough mother, wife, friend, employee, sister, ...?" We stress out about everything we are not doing well enough ... except for taking care of ourselves. We naturally feel guilty if we take time away from our other roles to focus on ourselves. It becomes a vicious circle because we don't feel strong and healthy, so we feel like we aren't performing any of our duties well. The truth is you will be better at everything in your life if you carve out just a few minutes in your day to focus on your health. Don't be overwhelmed! Start with small changes and as you grow stronger make more changes. I promise you will see results.

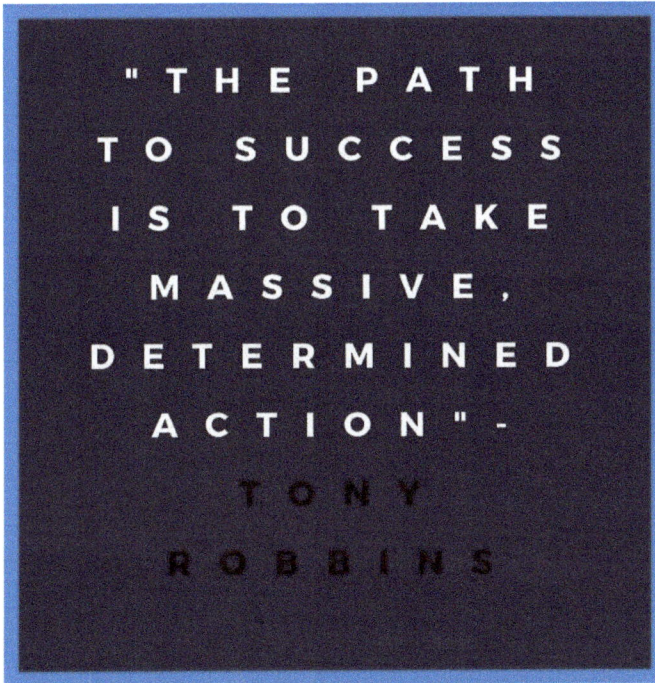

"THE PATH TO SUCCESS IS TO TAKE MASSIVE, DETERMINED ACTION" - TONY ROBBINS

Life is hard and it doesn't cut any of us any slack! You deserve to be the strongest version of yourself so that you can juggle all that your life throws at you. You deserve to feel good about yourself and enjoy the benefits of feeling strong and healthy. I talk to women who have achieved great weight loss to become healthy and those who only lost five or ten pounds to feel better, and they all have in common that they are incredibly proud of themselves! It takes a commitment to put priority on our own wellbeing - to adopt practices to take care of ourselves and not just others. And, once we make that commitment, it is an accomplishment that has positive effects in every aspect of our lives.

Here's another important first step that won't cost you anything: think about your relationship with food. What drives you when you make choices about what you put in your body? When do you eat and why? Food should be a source of nourishment and we should eat for survival, but too often we use food as a reward or for comfort from the stress of our daily lives. Many of us have developed an unhealthy relationship with food which has led to an unhealthy lifestyle. We eat in an attempt to treat or alleviate a host of bad feelings we may be experiencing such as stress, loneliness, boredom, unhappiness, etc. If this sounds familiar to you, start considering what motivates your diet choices and equip yourself to begin making healthy changes in what you eat and when you eat. This book is going to offer you some tools and options to get started.

We all know that the best life is one lived in balance and with moderation. Yes, you deserve a piece of cake at a birthday party or wedding. Yes, you deserve a scone over coffee with a friend or a girls' night with cocktails. Those are all wonderful parts of living, but you should be able to enjoy them guilt free.

Occasionally treating yourself to something you really want is part of a balanced lifestyle. If you treat yourself with poor choices every day, not only is it unbalanced but it will make you unhappy. Making better choices daily allows us to enjoy those special times with fewer worries or anxiety. Being healthy is not about a prescribed diet, it's about learning to live a healthy lifestyle that allows you to enjoy the best version of yourself!

You deserve good health and the chance to enjoy the pride that comes from watching yourself transform into a stronger, healthier woman. It takes planning and work, but it's guaranteed you will love the rewards. I want to challenge you to take the tools and suggestions in this book and begin making some changes that will lead to a better you. If your goal is a major transformation, it'll take a lot of work, but you'll be so proud of yourself for making the effort.

Are you ready to start feeling like the best version of yourself? Let's get started – what do you have to lose?

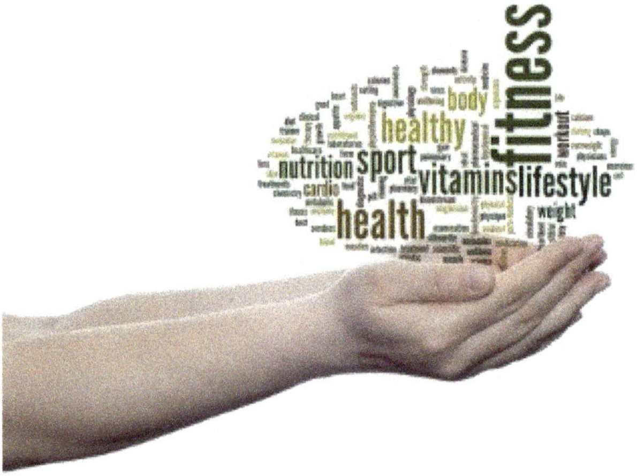
fitness
body
healthy
nutrition
sport
vitaminslifestyle
cardio
health
weight

Chapter 2 Staying Motivated

Let's talk about motivation for a bit – you'll enjoy this journey more if you plan sources of motivation along the way. Some changes are going to occur right away, but some will come more gradually. Some of us are more impatient than others, and when we become frustrated with our efforts not producing desirable results, we give up. Research tells us that once we start making healthier choices, we notice the effects in about two weeks. Those close to us notice in about four weeks, but people who don't see us daily won't notice for about six weeks. So, we need a plan for staying motivated when we aren't experiencing the euphoria of success. Here are a few suggestions to get started.

1. Always keep in mind what motivated you to begin your journey finding a better you. Many mothers will say they want to have the energy to play with their children. Some of us want the energy to do our job better or be a better partner for our significant other. And, let's face it: vanity is a great motivator. Some of us just want to look better. We want to feel attractive. Whenever you feel like sliding back into your comfortable bad habits, think about what first made you step up and take on the challenge to be better. You might not have reached your goal yet, but you are improving and getting

stronger every day. Change won't happen back there in the Comfort Zone.

2. Surround yourself with people and things that support your journey. Connect with friends and family who have similar goals and build a support system. Share recipes and exercise plans. A workout partner is a great help, even if you just take a walk together a few days a week. There are hundreds of inspirational bloggers to follow who offer motivation, recipes, and lifestyle advice. Find a few that you enjoy and interact with their blogs. You'll learn so much and the different choices you find will keep you from getting bored.

3. Use technology! Fitbits are fabulous devices to get started. You can connect with friends and engage in healthy competitions – compete to see who makes those 10,000 steps most often. It'll also track your sleeping patterns so that you can at least become aware of how much rest you are getting. There are also hundreds of apps to choose from to help you with every aspect of a healthy lifestyle. My Fitness Pal and Map My Fitness remain top-rated, but a search will render hundreds of excellent options, many for free! You can find apps that will help with recipes, music for your

workout, meditation tips, or even a prescribed workout. If you are stuck indoors, go to YouTube for an abundance of workout video choices for any exercise and any skill level.

4. Preparation is also a great motivator. If you prepare for the journey, you'll be much more successful and you'll enjoy the trip a lot more. Take a few minutes at the beginning of each week and make a menu. Stock your kitchen with healthy foods and lots of choices so you don't get bored. **Do not fill your grocery cart with bad processed foods!!** I hear women all the time say they have to keep snacks for their children and then they eventually give in to eating the processed snacks themselves. Don't buy the processed snacks! Your children's developing bodies do not need that unhealthy garbage either! This is a great time for you to set a good example and also to teach your children how to make healthy snack choices. Recipes abound for making quick kid-friendly snacks from whole foods. Make your journey a family affair. Your family might not be thrilled to join, but it certainly won't damage them.

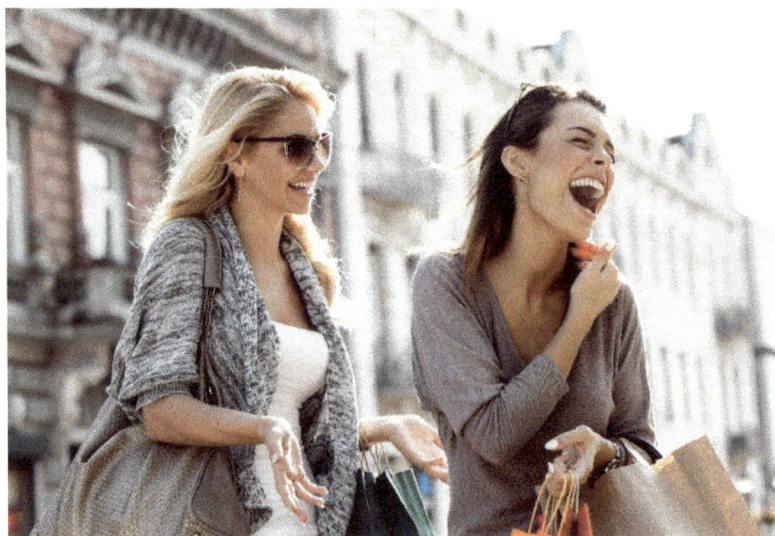

Honestly, we are all going to fail sometimes. That's part of life – it's part of learning. You are going to be making changes in many areas on your journey to better health, and it won't be healthy until you find the balance that makes you happy. You won't always be perfect, but your efforts are going to make you stronger. You'll be taking care of your physical and mental health, and you will be proud of the woman you find in the mirror.

Chapter 3 Diet --- Ugh

The word "diet" conjures those negative thoughts, I know. <u>It's because diets don't work.</u> They come with rules and all sorts of unrealistic expectations that we can't follow long-term. We naturally want to find a way to make them easy, to cheat. A healthy lifestyle means no need to cheat because you work to achieve a balance that you can maintain your whole life. Counting calories does not work because we automatically think we are being deprived. If you make good dietary choices from real whole foods, you won't need to count calories. You'll feel satisfied more easily even though you'll be eating less.

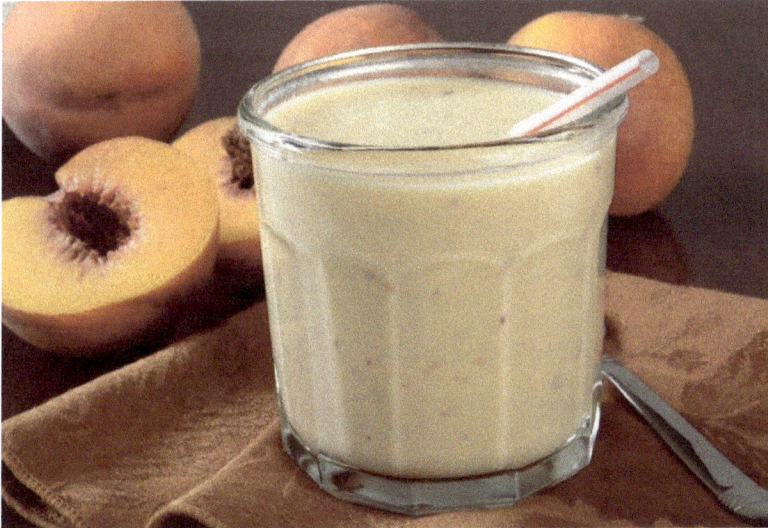

It can be overwhelming to consider a complete overhaul of our diet. Here is an adage that's helpful in getting started. It's from the late Dr. Annemarie Colbin who founded The Natural

Gourmet Institute: "If it doesn't run, fly, swim, or grow from the ground, it's not food." Don't worry about counting calories. Keep moderation in mind, but eat what you want of real food. Stay away from items with a long list of ingredients and most certainly stay away from ingredients you can't identify. Start being mindful about what you put in your body!

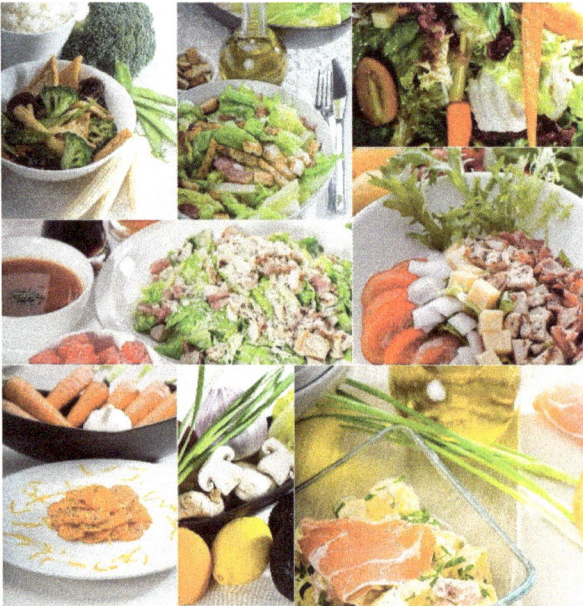

Build your meals around lean protein like chicken, turkey, seafood, eggs, nuts, venison, and lean beef (preferably grass fed) along with a variety of fruits and vegetables. Limit carbohydrates and eliminate processed food items and you'll experience amazing results quickly. Another essential is preparing and cooking most of your meals at home. At home you are completely in control of what ingredients you use and how you cook. When you do eat out, choose options that seem the least processed.

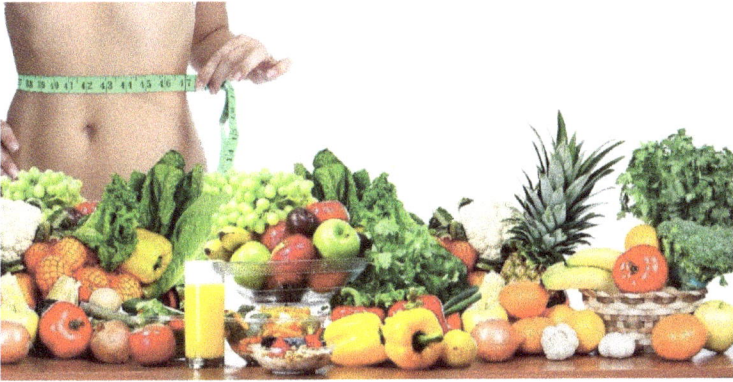

I would like to say there is a way to avoid the work and still be healthy, but alas I am afraid there is not. A healthy, balanced life is going to mean you spend some time planning for what you will eat, shopping for it, and then cooking it at home. I know, I know – we all work hard and we like for somebody to serve us and wait on us once in a while. This is a challenge for most of us, and it will really test your commitment on this journey to a healthier lifestyle. Nothing wrong with a luncheon or night out to socialize and unwind, but as with every other part of life, we have to keep moderation in mind. The majority of meals need to be prepared in your own kitchen. I promise you'll soon feel better and you'll be proud of your efforts!

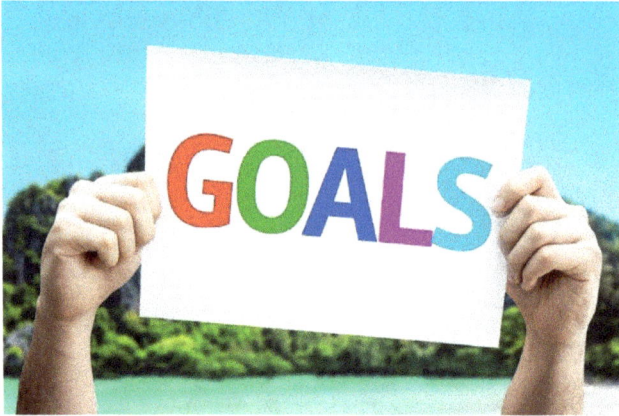

What this book offers you is not a prescribed diet, but some tips to acquire a healthier diet along with some suggestions that will help you avoid some of the pitfalls that might stymie your best results.

The first step to cleaning up your diet is cleaning out your kitchen! No matter how tempted you are to hoard those processed items that have a shelf-life of forever, don't do it. If you can't stand the thought of them going to waste, donate them to a local food bank. Let's consider some guidelines, tips, and suggestions for how to get rid of those items in your kitchen that are holding you back and leading to unhealthy habits.

1. Read labels! I'm warning you that you will be horrified at first when you realize what you've been putting in

your body. Just because the packaging proclaims the item as healthy, does not mean it is. Many of the products well-known as "healthy" or "diet" are processed and preserved and contain high levels of sugar and salt --- and who knows what else. We can't even pronounce or identify most of what has been added to what might have once been something edible. They might be low in calories, but they are not beneficial to overall health. Stay away from items with genetically modified organism (GMO) ingredients. The jury is still out and the battle is still on about the effects of altering the genetic makeup of our food, but what is certain is nobody is sure what harm this stuff is really doing our bodies. It is a complex issue and it deserves your time. If you haven't read up on GMO's, you should do so and make decisions about what you are willing to accept in your diet. The best way to start eliminating these items is to look for "organic" or "non-GMO Project Verified" labels. Buy dairy and meats that are "grass fed" or "caught wild".   Look for produce labeled "vine ripened". Try it, and you'll be amazed how much better you feel.

2. Now, let's get the skinny on sugar: It's sweet goodness that we all need. The problem is we ingest way more

than we need, and we typically have no idea how much or how often we put it in our bodies. The harmful effects of too much processed sugar would be another topic that really deserves your research. Being aware that it hides almost anywhere and realizing the negative effects of a sugary diet will be great motivation to clean it out. Here is an example for gauging your intake. The American Heart Association recommends women have 24 grams of sugar a day. About four teaspoons of sugar is equal to 1 gram. A brand name low-calorie/ low-fat container of yogurt has 18 grams of sugar. What you thought was a healthy snack, contains almost your entire daily recommended allowance of sugar. And, that soft drink you treated yourself with contains approximately 40 grams of sugar (some contain more). Now, who really has just one serving of a soft drink? They are bottled as 2 ½ servings. That's roughly 100 grams of sugar – WOW! Ever try munching on 25 teaspoons of sugar as a snack? – Bleh! Chances are if a product is labeled "low fat", sugar has replaced the fat and it isn't any healthier. Read labels and be aware of how much you are actually eating. We all need a little sweetness in our lives, but too much is going to leave us feeling sick and unhappy. Go for healthier options like stevia, or munch on some fresh fruits. You can also use some honey or maple syrup. Occasional coconut or brown or cane sugar is also fine.

3. Stock your kitchen with fresh herbs and spices to replace salt. Even those of us who appear healthy can be damaging our bodies with too much salt. Guidelines recommend 1500 mg (3.75gm) – 2300 mg (6gm) of sodium a day for the average adult. Too much sodium has been proven to lead to heart disease, high blood pressure, stroke, kidney failure, and an assortment of other ailments. Salt is another ingredient that hides everywhere as a preservative. Those frozen "diet" entrées you pop in the microwave at lunch can have over 900 mg of sodium. Read labels to make sure you aren't ingesting your daily allowance in one meal. You'll find that seasoning food with a variety of other fresh herbs and spices will eliminate the need for salt as flavoring. If you retain water like most women do, salt will exacerbate the problem and make you appear bloated and heavier than you really are. Many women also report that they do not feel as hungry during the day once they reduce sodium intake. Many of us don't realize that the table salt we add to our food is actually processed and contains harmful chemicals. Look for ways to eliminate or replace salt in your diet. Sea salt

or Himalayan salt are better options because they are natural non-iodized and do have some health benefits ... when used in moderation.

4. If your goal is significant weight-loss, go gluten-free. Even if you don't experience full-blown allergic reactions to it, any sensitivity to it can hinder your weight-loss efforts. The truth is we all feel better without it, and it is in almost all processed foods. Plus, when you eliminate gluten, it forces you to choose whole foods in their natural form. Gluten is another item you need to educate yourself on so that you can make smarter choices in your diet. Research has proven that gluten-free / low- carb is the best diet for significant weight-loss. To learn more about gluten-free diets, I recommend you check out this blog where they offer a free eBook (healthy desserts, yum!) as a welcome gift:

www.kiraglutenfreerecipes.com

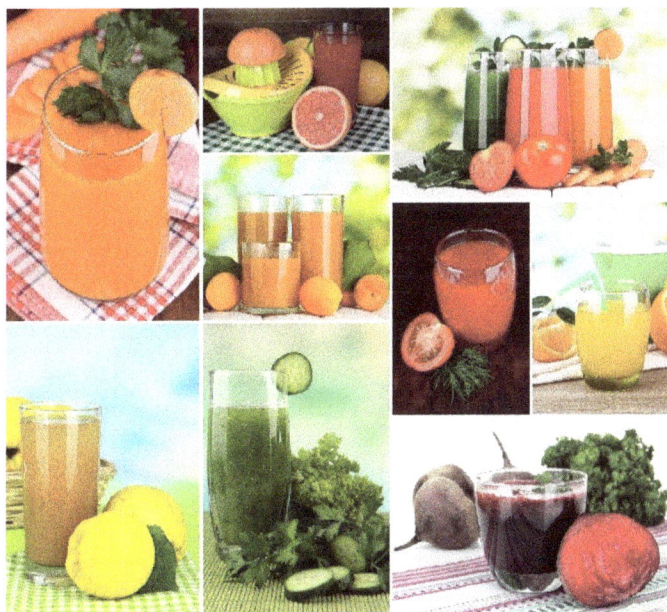

5. Stock up on superfoods and replace your less than healthy temptations with nutrient-rich foods that improve health and wellbeing. Some that have recently garnered superfood status are kale, spinach, broccoli, Brussel sprouts, blueberries, sweet potatoes, pomegranates, quinoa, salmon, almonds, ... Whew! Those are just a few to choose from. Kale (and most other leafy greens) provides more antioxidants than most other veggies, and along with broccoli and Brussel sprouts, it has detoxification powers that help your liver eliminate toxic by- products from your other not-so-healthy food choices. Kale is extra super because you

can eat it raw, saute it, broil it, steam it, or add it to a smoothie. Blueberries are also chock full off antioxidants, fiber, and Vitamin C. Pomegranates are also now being lauded for their cancer-fighting potential and proven ability to boost immunity. Sweet potatoes are rich in beta-carotene, potassium, and fiber, and are always considered a healthy tubular option. The Omega-3 fatty acids and amino acids in salmon boast a variety of health benefits that include decreased blood pressure and cholesterol, better vision, and repaired nerve damage. Winter squash is an excellent source of both beta-carotene and Omega-3's, along with the fiber that helps to fill you up. Chickpeas are another popular superfood. They are very low in fat and sodium, high in protein, iron, vitamins, fiber, and antioxidants. Mash them with some olive oil and herbs to make humus you enjoy with some broccoli or cauliflower for a super tasty and nutrient-rich snack! These are only a few superfood options, so you should definitely research and find some nutrient-rich foods you can add to your table. Enjoy these selections as a side or in a salad, soup, or smoothie. Think of it as using food as medicine. Don't cheat yourself! Start experiencing the benefits of these super powers in your diet! You can also recommend with powdered super foods such as chlorella, spirulina, or barley grass.

Alfalfa is also fantastic and it helps alkalize and detoxify the body.

6. Use only unsaturated or "good" fats. Not all fats are bad. Monounsaturated and polyunsaturated fats benefit heart health and insulin levels. They can make you feel full and curb cravings for "bad" fats that carry a variety of harmful effects for our bodies. Some good sources of unsaturated fats include unrefined olive oil and coconut oil, flaxseed oil, grapeseed oil, and nuts. Avocados and non-GMO tofu are other excellent choices of "good" fats. Almonds and walnuts are great sources of "good" fat and protein, so just a palm full can make you feel full and curb cravings. Try making condiments with these bases and flavored vinegars and lemon and lime juice. Remember moderation is the key to becoming healthier, so it is important to stay within the recommended daily allowance. The recommendation for women is that 20% - 35% of daily calories come from healthy sources of fat.

You are what you drink ... so, let's talk about that

None of us need an expert to tell us that the best drink is purified water and we should be drinking plenty of it. You don't have to look far to find the research supporting the detrimental effects of soft drinks and diet sodas. Diet sodas are a chemical cocktail that should never be considered a healthy choice. Fruit and vegetable juices can be processed with added sugar and sodium until the nutritional value is out the window. As a matter of fact, you'll find your grocery store shelves full of choices claiming to be healthy drinks, but read the labels and you'll find an assortment of ingredients that are anything but. So, what do we drink? Sometimes we need a little flavor and a little comfort from our daily liquid choices. A good guideline is to think of drinks the way we think of food. Consider what nutritional value it offers.

1. Purified water is always the best choice. Adding some lemon or lime is adding some taste and nutritional value. Another healthy option is to fill the bottom of your glass with fresh fruits and add ice and water – healthy and refreshing. If you really enjoy fruit juice, cut it in half with water for a lighter option that won't be so harsh on your body. Water is always our best drink choice and we need 6-8 8 ounce servings a day to reap all its benefits.

2. The subject of coffee is a murky one, indeed. One report will praise its super powers while another will warn of it catastrophic effects. Again, the key here is moderation. If it is a must in your life, one to two cups a day seems to be the recommendation in order to experience its benefits and none of its harm. Unfortunately, not only do we tend to drink too much of it, we tend to add a lot of sugary and fatty flavor to it that ends up making something natural another chemical cocktail we swallow down. Drinking it black, either hot or over ice, is best; but if you need flavor, try coconut or almond milk as creamer --- fewer calories and just as much flavor.

3. Tea is an excellent option that you can sip on throughout your day. A warm mug on chilly days can provide that same comfort you get from coffee, and green tea and chai tea are antioxidants packed with nutritional value. Sip some green tea hot or over ice and you'll feel energized and more alert. Its medicinal value has also been linked to both heart disease and cancer prevention. Chai tea has been found to support digestion, prevent cancer, lower blood sugar and promote cardiovascular health. It also contains anti-inflammatory agents that give it medicinal properties as well. You are going to find your grocery shelves

abounding with varieties of both these popular teas – every flavor imaginable has been concocted. Be sure to read labels and make certain you are buying natural forms. Just like with food choices, if you can't identify the ingredients, let it go.

4. Here's another murky topic: alcohol consumption. Clearly we all know the hazards of consuming too much – clearly the topic of another book - let's just look at it from the perspective of diet and feeling healthier. Research will say it makes you fat and research will say it can help you lose weight. It might cause cardiovascular problems or it might improve cardiovascular health. The issue is that it affects each of us differently, so the magic word again is "moderation." Moderation for women is considered one drink a day or no more than 6 – 8 drinks a week. If your goal is to lose weight, it's best to eliminate alcohol or make low calorie choices. Even if the alcohol we consume isn't adding pounds, it tends to lower our inhibitions, so we eat more than we might normally consume. It also causes us to retain water that will hang around for days! If you want to drink moderately, continue to choose lower calorie options like lite beer, vodka with tonic water, or red wine which is proven to have a variety of health benefits when enjoyed in moderation. Avoid adding

mixes and fruit juices that are full of sugar, sodium, and harmful chemicals.

More tips for natural weight loss drinks:

Start juicing vegetables and leafy greens. Invest in a quality juicer, like Omega Juicer.

Treat yourself to one nutritious vegetable juice a day. The best juicing recipes for weight loss include cucumbers, fennel, spinach, beets, tomatoes and ginger. You can season your juices with some Himalayan salt to taste. Keep hydrated and nicely energized!

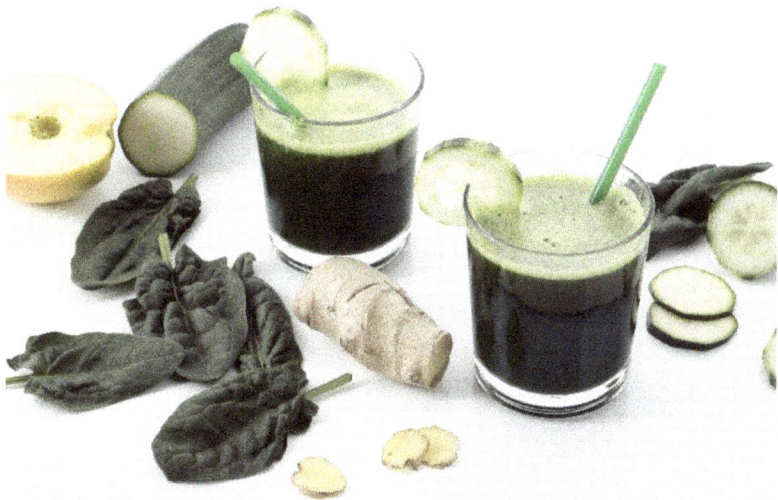

"The body is like a piano, and happiness is like music. It is needful to have the instrument in good order."

Henry Ward Beecher (1813 – 1887)

Ah, how to keep the body in good order when you are trying to keep everything else in good order? It's a challenge for sure, and this is where those of us with even the best intentions often give up on realizing our potential to be strong, healthy women. This is also where that image of a tall, thin supermodel that we will never be squashes our efforts to be the best that we can be. Exercise shouldn't be about making you skinny; it should be about making you strong. It should be about fine tuning you into the best instrument you can be. We let ourselves get discouraged by our failures to reach unrealistic expectations and we give up on the process that could be so beneficial to our overall health. Exercise and physical activity are essential for a happy, healthy lifestyle.

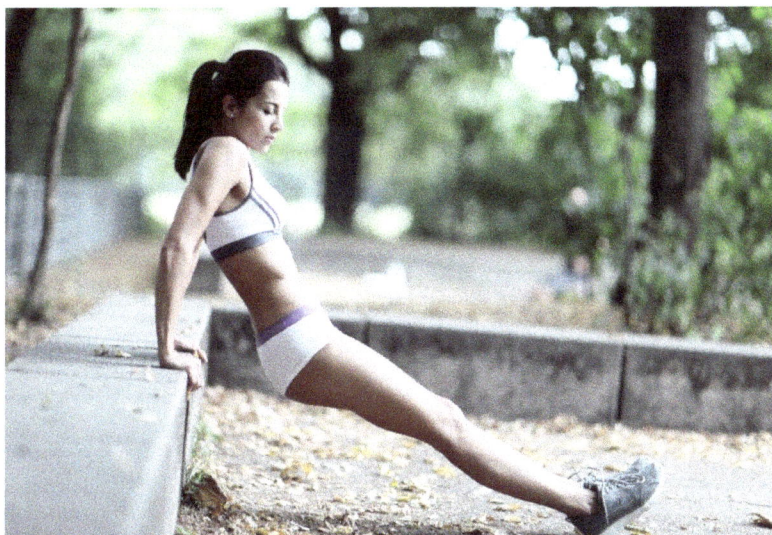

Consider these benefits to an active lifestyle: Exercise makes you happier – really, it does! Exercise is like a <u>free antidepressant</u>. It's been proven to reduce stress and anxiety, plus relieve depression and sleep deprivation. You'll have more energy during the day and sleep better at night. You'll be proud of even the small milestones that you reach, and that pride will make you more confident in other areas of your life. Research is revealing that regular exercise is also instrumental in preventing Alzheimer's and dementia. It's not just important to our physical health, it's essential for maintaining our mental health as well.

 If that isn't enough motivation, consider that it significantly improves your sex life. That's right. Regular exercise not only gives you more energy for a healthy sex life, it also improves your appearance and self-esteem making you feel more desirable. A good workout triggers endorphins and adrenaline that boost your vitality, desire, and capacity for sexual activity. Get your partner on board for regular exercise and workout together. You'll enjoy double benefits!

"My job is to be fit and I'm really blessed that I get to go and work out and live a really healthy lifestyle."- Kerri Walsh

Here's more motivation – regular exercise is a major part of taking care of yourself so that you can effectively and successfully perform all the other duties in your busy life. Our bodies are not meant for the sedentary lifestyle we have created. The body is a huge muscle that needs to be constantly stretched and toned. The heart and lungs are muscles that will atrophy if we don't use them to their capacity. You should do something every day that gets your heart rate up and causes you to breathe deeply. Don't wait for the day when you think it might come easily for you. That day won't come and you'll never realize how strong you really are.

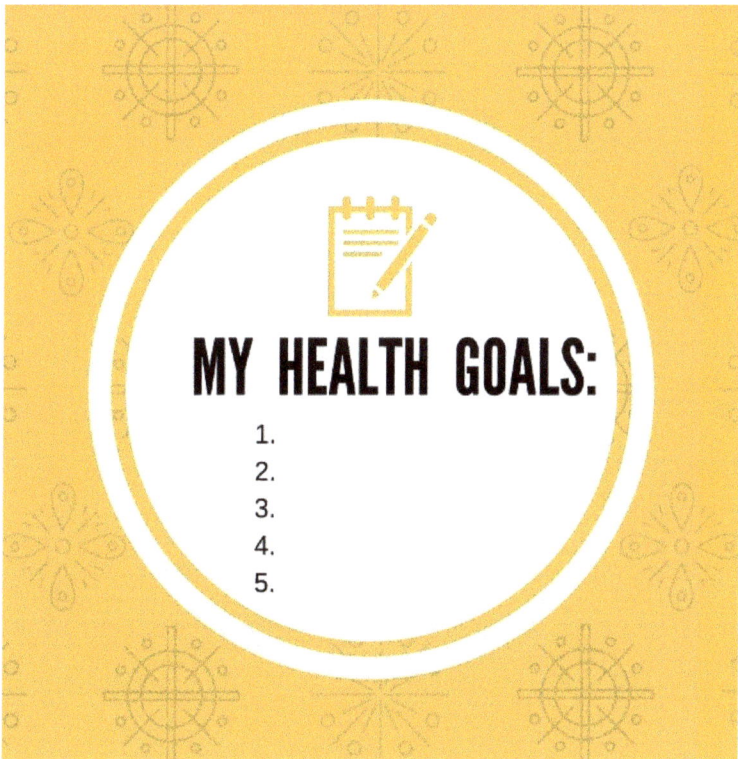

MY HEALTH GOALS:

1.
2.
3.
4.
5.

So, how do you get started leading a more active lifestyle? Just like you did with your diet, consider where you are right now and plan where you can make changes to include more physical activity in your day. How many days a week do you exercise now? Are you leading a completely sedentary lifestyle? Are you active but need to add muscle tone to become stronger? Have you ever practiced a regular exercise program? Think about what motivated you to consider becoming more physically active. Do you want to look better? Feel better? Enjoy improved health? Now, make some short-term and long-term goals and let's get started! <u>You deserve to feel well and strong!</u>

No matter where you are on the fitness spectrum, you can add some physical activity that will help you lead a healthier life. Think about it like this – fit women are not in the gym working to get skinny and attractive; they are in the gym maintaining their healthy beautiful bodies. There won't be a day when all your goals are met and you can quit exercising. You have to commit to it as an essential part of your overall healthier life. It's extremely important that you find an activity you enjoy, so that daily exercise doesn't feel like another chore. Find an activity that produces beneficial emotional effects for you as well as physical. If you feel good about doing it, you'll be more likely to make it a habit.

If your lifestyle is currently pretty sedentary, ease into activities that you find enjoyable and increase duration and intensity as you become stronger. Many of us self-sabotage right away because we try programs and routines that are too difficult for our current fitness level. We injure ourselves or our muscles are so sore we can't function for a few days, so once we recover we don't want to go back to whatever it was. You'll experience more long-term success if you ease into an exercise program that you enjoy.

The best routine for women to experience a real transformation in their bodies is a combination of cardio and weight training. The American Heart Association recommends 30 minutes of cardiovascular activity a day. The Center for Disease Control recommends 150 minutes a week. Now, if you aren't ready for 30 minutes, do what you can! If you are beginning and you need to start with 15 minutes, you'll soon find yourself capable of 30 minutes and more. You'll be building a habit that will render great rewards.

Chapter 4 Carving time for Cardio

Most of us lead such busy lives we really don't have time for a gym membership or a personal trainer. And, let's be honest, if you are out of shape or not feeling confident about your skill level, gyms are intimidating. So, how do we fit in 30 minutes to an hour for cardio in every day? Walking, jogging, biking, gardening, swimming, and dancing are all great aerobic activities that can be done with family and friends. If you are having trouble getting started, consider your daily activities and find where one of these would naturally fit.

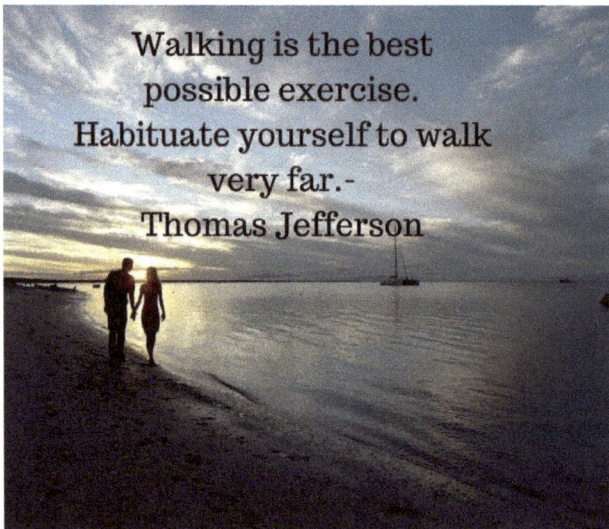

Walking is the best possible exercise. Habituate yourself to walk very far. - Thomas Jefferson

Some of us have to make the commitment to rising 30 minutes earlier and getting it in before we start our day. If that's not an option, think about times in your day when you are sedentary and consider how you could fill those minutes with exercise. Taking the baby or your dog for a walk or jog in the afternoon would have great benefits for all. If you are shuttling kids to sports practices, take a 30 -minute walk or jog while you wait. Most practices are an hour, so you'll still have time to watch Jr. kick the soccer ball around, and you might find other moms joining you. It won't take long and you'll be walking a little longer, a little farther, and a little faster.

If you watch television in the evening, don't be a couch potato! Find ways to break a sweat while you catch up on *Grey's Anatomy!* They have televisions in gyms for a reason; working out can be boring and watching is a good distraction. You will probably find that you exercise longer because you are engrossed in whatever show you are watching. Keep your workout equipment near the television and pull it out while you watch. Use dumbbells, resistance bands, or a medicine ball and strength train. Or, jog in place, do crunches, jumping jacks, leg lifts, toe touches, or lunges. Break a sweat!

Another good activity to get started is dancing. Can't make it to a Zumba class? Turn on your favorite playlist and dance around the house while you complete some of your evening chores. You don't see many dancers who aren't in shape because it's difficult and it burns calories. Fit Radio is a popular free app that provides playlists in a variety of genres geared toward exercise. Buying a premium package allows you to make your own lists, but the free lists are great for beginners. Challenge yourself to dance through a whole list or a certain number of songs. Pretty soon you'll be ready for a more challenging activity.

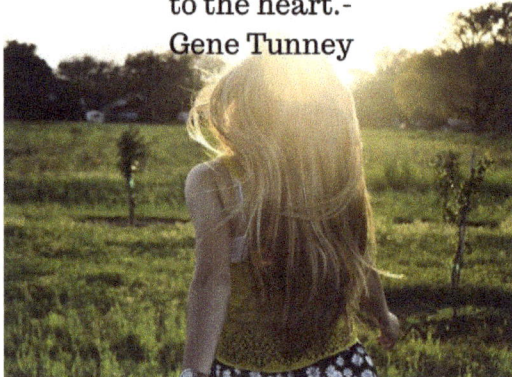

Exercise should be regarded as tribute to the heart.- Gene Tunney

Here's another idea – turn on your computer! YouTube abounds with workout videos for everybody. You can find the 4-minute, 7-minute, and 10- minute workout sequence for almost any activity at any skill level. Full workouts for strength training and full-body cardio are right at your fingertips. Of course, you'll want to research and make sure they are produced by experts, but plenty feature popular renowned fitness experts with years of experience. It's like having a professional trainer in your home at your convenience. And, as we mentioned earlier, if it exists, there's an app for it. Many of the fitness apps available allow you to choose the type of exercise you need and then customize your routine ...FOR FREE! Use the technology you have available to help you get started moving during the day.

Chapter 5 Building Muscle

For decades we've been skipping out on weight training by using the excuse that we don't want to bulk up and look manly. So, we've been missing out on the benefits of a toned body with lean muscle mass. Women don't typically have the hormones required to pack on bulky muscle, so unless you are planning to take supplements and train like a bodybuilder, you needn't worry about a few hours a week lifting light weights turning you into The Hulk. Plus, we all have to admit we envy those women who are a little bit older and are still looking good in tanks and sleeveless blouses. We'd all like to look more toned and confident.

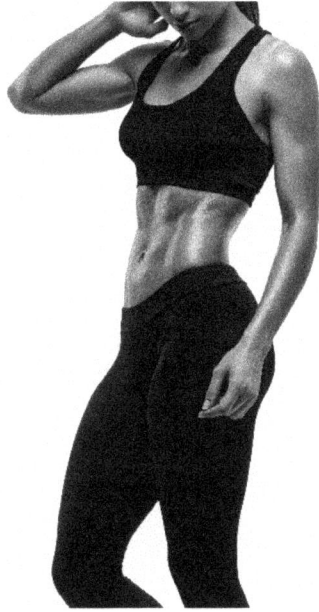

If you really want to transform your body and get stronger, you'll have to hit the weights. It's recommended for women to strength train for 20-30 minutes 2-3 days a week. However, whatever time you can get in is going to be very beneficial to your overall health and appearance, and you do not need a gym membership to get started. Toned muscle burns fat and calories. You'll burn more calories and your body will look leaner than it will if you stick to just cardio workouts. Also, a little strength training helps us maintain our posture and fight Osteoporosis. The good news is we can build muscle as long as we live, so it's never too late to start.

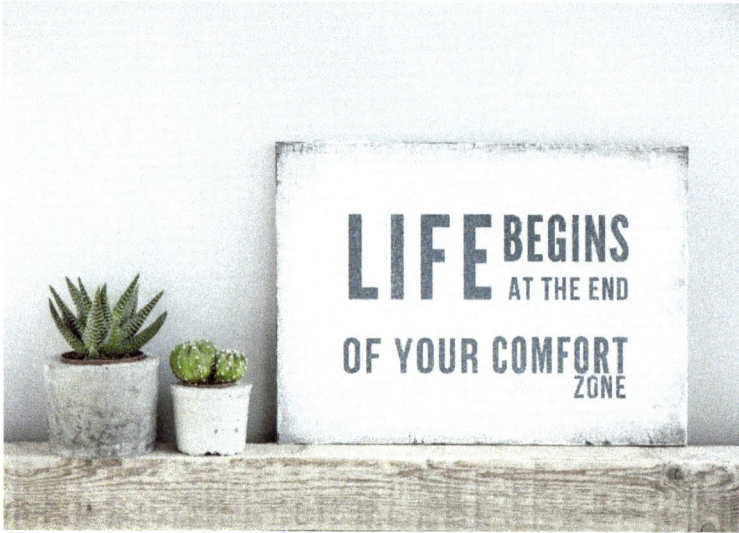

Start with weights light enough that you can complete sets of 12-15 repetitions. It won't take long before you'll be ready to move to heavier weights and try adding new moves. Dumbbells are perfect for getting started, but resistance bands, medicine balls, or kettle balls are great choices too. These often come with instructions for suggested exercises and routines. If you aren't ready for any of those, do the recommended reps using soup cans. If you follow through, you'll be surprised at how quickly you will feel confident enough to increase the weight. I promise – you'll see results and you'll like what you see.

Chapter 6 Exercising Your Soul

If there is anything we women fail to take care of more than our bodies, it's our minds. Our day is filled with rushing from place to place, solving problems at home and at work, caring for others, and then dealing with our own burdens and emotional baggage. Who can keep up with it all? We lie down at night with our mind still spinning with the problems of the day, so then we don't sleep well. We wake up still physically and emotionally fatigued and ill-equipped to deal with the next day's drama – another vicious circle that becomes our life.

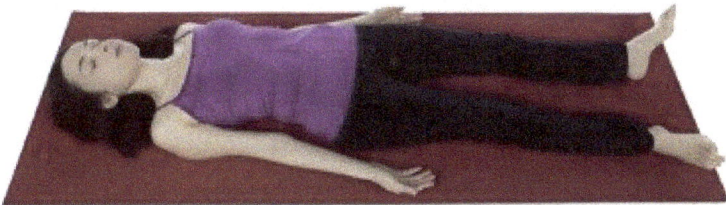

As important as it is to clean the toxins from our bodies, it's even more important to clean them from our mind. The good news is it really only takes minutes to let go of negative thoughts and clear the junk from your head. Practicing just a few minutes of some type of quiet time or meditation will decrease stress and anxiety, help you sleep, and increase your spiritual connection.

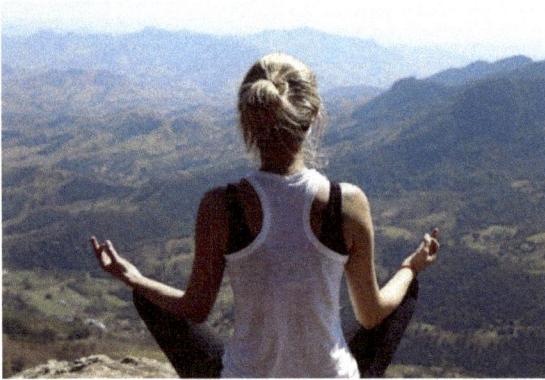

The problem is we don't like silence. We are afraid of silence, so we strive to fill up every second of our lives with noise. We often express the need for quiet, but when given the chance we don't take it. We seek out noise to fill the emptiness. Taking just a few minutes to silence your mind gives it a chance to renew and create order out of the chaos of the day. It's a way to nourish your soul, and taking time to do it will make you so much more productive in every part of your life. It takes practice and it takes commitment.

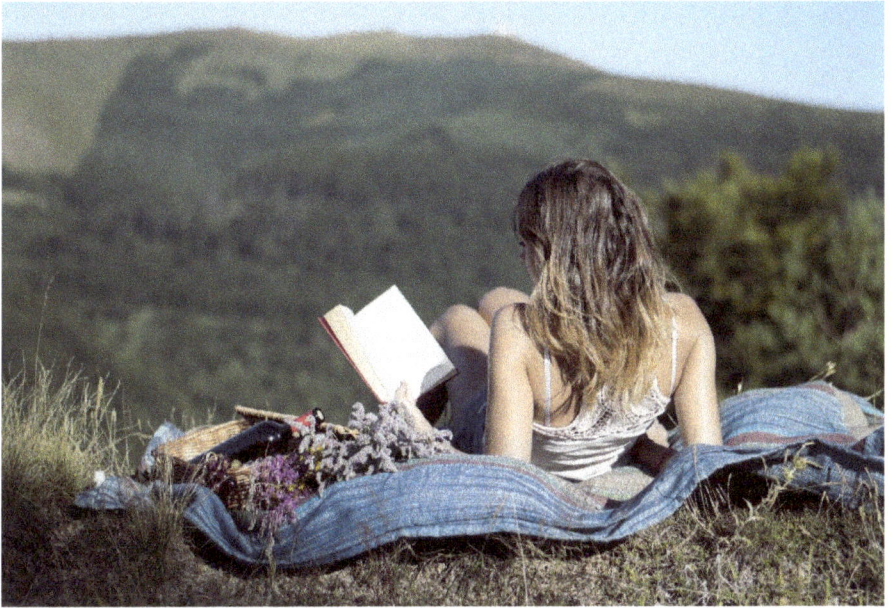

Society is so fast paced and we are so bombarded by constant images and noises, it's hard to find the time and place to be alone and refresh. If you feel your life is too hectic to find quiet, start by committing just 2-3 minutes a day. Once you experience the amazing effects of what you find in quiet, you'll begin making more time to renew your mind and spirit.

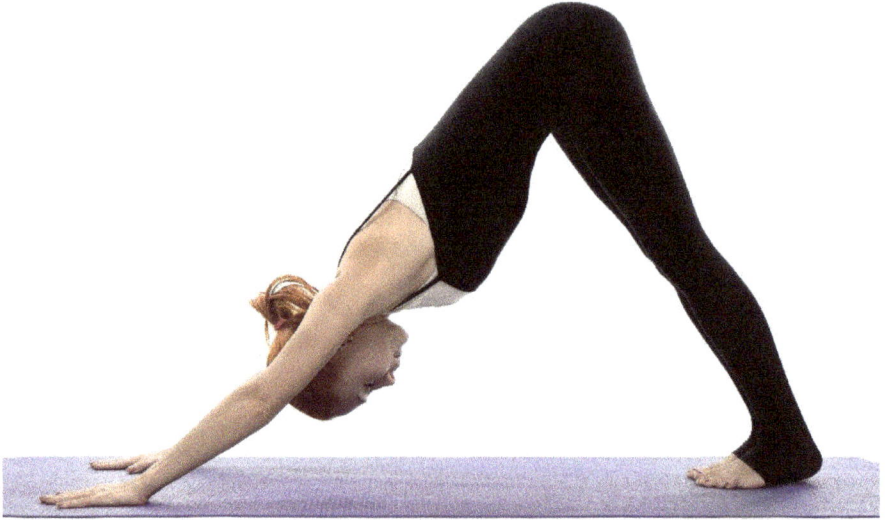

It can also be a little naturally overwhelming to commit to doing nothing, but it's so important for our body and soul. It's a prescribed therapy for those who seek mental health counseling because it allows us to center and really find ourselves when we get lost in the chaos of life. Some planning before you get started can ensure it's an enjoyable and successful experience.

1. Plan a place – I know, easier said than done. But, it can be done. Think of somewhere you are most comfortable that is accessible every day – somewhere free from distraction. Many women immediately choose the bathtub – nothing like a warm bath! Other suggestions

are a place outdoors, a sauna, your favorite chair, wherever you feel relaxed.

2. Schedule a time. You'll be more likely to commit if you view it as an appointment. If you only have 2-3 minutes to spare for silent breathing, start there. Anytime you give yourself to slow down and center will be helpful to your overall wellbeing.

3. Decide what you hope to accomplish from the time you spend. Do you need to calm yourself down after a hectic day? Do you want a stronger spiritual connection? Do you need relaxation for better sleep? Do you need a better sense of self? Thinking about what your needs are can help you plan a method for meditation.

4. Here's the most important: Decide how you want to spend this time. If you have no idea where to start, practice deep breathing. Maybe you need to spend it in prayer. Many people find peace in repeating a positive phrase in their head like a mantra while forcing all other thoughts out. Yoga is a wonderful practice that exercises the body and soul. If you've never tried it, you should. Do some research and you'll find plenty of

beginner sessions online. It can be practiced without any equipment and effective sessions can only take minutes. It's a beautiful practice that makes you feel strong and confident.

However you choose to spend this time, make sure you are as disciplined about it as you are exercising your body. Don't feel guilty about taking a few minutes to renew your mind. It is just as important to your health and it's an integral part of taking care of ourselves.

Chapter 7 Sleep, Where Art Thou?

Six to eight hours of sleep a night is recommended for women. We all know that very few of us get enough sleep to be healthy and productive. We all have our personal demons that haunt us at night and keep sleep at bay. However, most women discover that once they take the time to take care for themselves and begin balancing their lives, sleeping patterns are greatly improved. To be honest, we all know that sleep issues are very complex and can be multifactorial. Some issues that deprive us of sleep are hormone related and some stem from diagnosed medical problems.

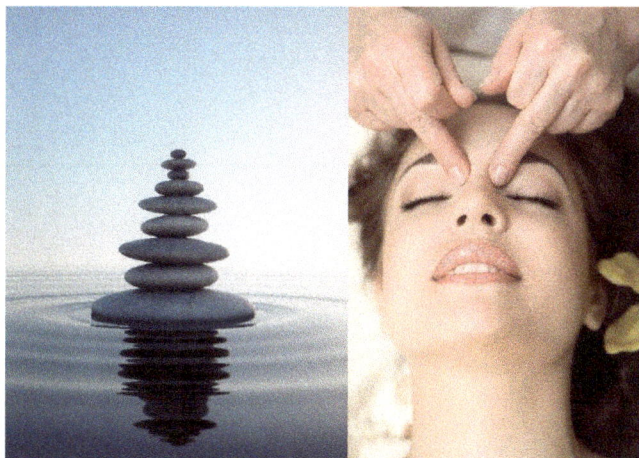

But, some can be regulated with lifestyle changes. Exercising to tire your body and then practicing deep breathing to relax it can be very effective. Once you begin living a lifestyle filled with healthy food, daily exercise and activity, and meditation, you'll be amazed at how easily sleep will come. Proper sleep and rest are so important for a happy, fulfilled life. Take care of yourself and make sure you give yourself enough sleep. If you feel you need help, seek it! It's part of taking control of your own wellbeing.

Closing

The journey toward a better self is a life journey. Once these new choices become habits, it'll be an easy road to follow. You'll feel so good about yourself and you'll want to continue experiencing all the benefits of a balanced, healthy life. Don't think of these practices as a means-to-an-end. They should become habits in your life that lead to a new more enjoyable lifestyle.

Decide today that you want to discover just how awesome you can be! Take the suggestions here that will help you and begin taking care of your physical, mental, and spiritual health. Love yourself and take responsibility for your own wellbeing. You deserve to be happy, fit, and strong!

To your success + enjoy the process!

Elena Garcia

PS. Before I go, I need to ask you a favor. If you received any value from this book, could you please rank it on Amazon and post an honest review?

Even one sentence will do.

I am always very excited to hear from my readers and your review can inspire other women to change their lifestyles, to get health and energy they deserve.

Thank You!

You can also reach me via email at:

elenajamesbooks@gmail.com